STUDIOS

T A L M A

Read also:
– *Prayers of Healing of the Yellow Emperor* (07/2024).

Disclaimer. The content of this book is not intended to be a substitute for professional medical advice, diagnosis or treatment. Always consult with a qualified and licensed physician or other medical care provider, and follow their advice without delay regardless of anything read in this book. Under no circumstance shall we have any liability to you for any loss or damage of any kind incurred as a result of the use of this book. Your use of it is at your own risk.

ISBN: 978-1-913191-44-3

Talma Studios International
Clifton House, Fitzwilliam St Lower,
Dublin 2 – Ireland
info@talmastudios.com
www.talmastudios.com

Amaya Chu Shen

PRAYERS OF LIFE

OF THE YELLOW EMPEROR

Translated from French

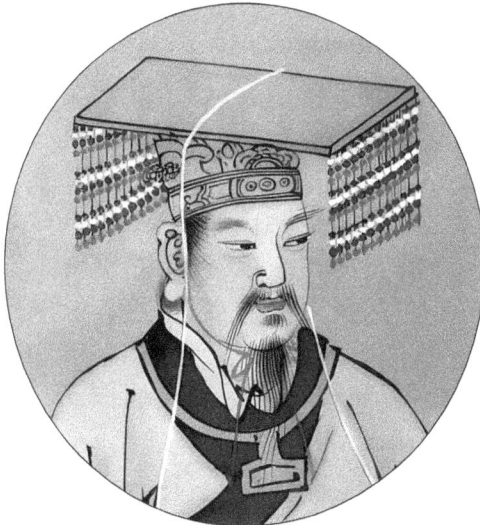

STUDIOS
TALMA

Presentation

Every era sees the appearance of exceptional beings. This is especially true in the realm of health. So why not attempt to connect with them? Why not attempt to bring the light of their knowledge to humanity, even long after they have departed?

Certainly, this endeavor may seem foolish to minds confined by their own reason, but why not take the leep when the stakes are the well-being of humanity itself?

Hildegard of Bingen (1098-1179) stood out predominantly. Though her name is little known to the general public, she ranks among the most fascinating figures of all time. This is evidenced, amongst other things, by her works that establish her as the first European naturopath in history. Communication flowed smoothly, but she informed us that her time had come to an end.

Then, our choice eagerly turned to the Yellow Emperor (黄帝 – Huangdi), the first of the five legendary emperors who lived in the 3rd millennium BC, revered as the father of Chinese civilization. Major works are attributed to him, including *Four Canons of the Yellow Emperor* (黃帝四經), but most importantly, concerning our aim of obtaining universal health, the *Huangdi Neijing* (黄帝内经) or the *Inner Canon of the Yellow Emperor*, which lays the foundation for traditional Chinese medicine. Indeed, Huangdi is its presumed creator.

As surprising as it may seem, "he" responded to us. What proof do we have that it was indeed him? The answer is self-evident: "none." Simply because we are not operating within the realm of scientific research, where experiments must be replicated under the same conditions to obtain the same result. Moreover, what interests us is the outcome, not the explanation, as it transcends us. Furthermore, the situation is easy to grasp as it unfolds in three acts: firstly, we asked a being, who departed from this world millennia ago, to aid humanity in matters of health; secondly, we received answers and thirdly, we share them.

They arrived in various forms, including the following *Prayers of Life of the Yellow Emperor*. We did not specifically request them, as our initial question was simply: "Yellow Emperor, can you help humanity get better?" As you will discover, they encompass other themes besides health and are not religious in nature, as they do not glorify Huangdi, who is never invoked within them.

We tested them on ourselves first. Then, our loved ones tried them before we offered them to the public. Regardless, we did not include their testimonies. We consider them worthless for the reader because only personal experience counts in this matter. Indeed, if such a prayer worked for a certain person in certain circumstances (besides, who can assert that it is truly the reason?), results are not guaranteed for anyone or on any subject. Consequently, it is not worth the consideration of abandoning your medical treatments and usual care, especially since we are not asking you to believe... We are simply recounting the initiated process and sharing these prayers as they came to us. It is up to each of you to discover them and decide how to use them.

Finally, know that these exchanges came with magical moments, indescribable emotions, and inexplicable synchronicities. More than anything, beyond the benefits that these prayers may bring to you, our deepest wish if for this wonderful world to illuminate your life.

Patrick Pasin
Publisher

P. S. Except for footnotes, the following words come from the Yellow Emperor (at least the being whom we addressed known by that name for five millennia), including the categorization of themes, the order of prayers, the explanations… everything. As for punctuation, don't be surprised: he wished for it to be minimal.

We also asked him to write an introduction. What could be more "normal," right? Now, may everything begin.

Introduction

We are all blessed with extrasensory abilities. We all possess the ability to aid in healing through the power of intention or prayer.

Stripped of its religious aspect, prayer is a powerful way of consciously connecting to energies. Words release bubbles of meaning and symbols, to reach the depths of the soul.

This directed thought calls upon all that is good, and hope is its vector of determination. It is hope that allows perseverance, the gathering of energies at a single point of deliverance.

Recollection, the deep journey into oneself, is necessary, for it is within that the sacred fire of understanding of Life burns.

Throughout history, shamans, sorcerers, druids have accompanied their healing with the sacred Word to infuse strength into their practices.

Precious and extraordinary, these prayers are allies.

They empower every person to commit to the well-being of humanity, an altruistic attitude that frees the ego from its veils of ephemeral satisfactions.

Each prayer that is spoken with conviction will carry the certainty that the Universe will offer what is most just to the person, as a messenger using its wings. And we must have the wisdom to accept what is.

It is within this mutual trust that miracles are born.

The Yellow Emperor

Pray

When seeking help from a prayer, it is essential to direct intention. Firstly, it is necessary to mentally focus on the subject or area to be addressed (if it's about healing), meaning to think directly about where one is suffering. Additionally, it is not enough to merely read the words that are written: it is by reading in a repetitive loop that they take effect. Chant them joyfully. They also gain in power if uttered with depth and genuine intention of obtaining the "healing" of the body or mind.

It is important to maintain a thought that is related to the request throughout the day. One can recite the prayer, but we can also use other means to keep the thread. That is why it is interesting to create a dedicated space at home where one can place the prayer, a photo of oneself or the person for whom the request is for, candles, or any other object symbolizing this continuum and the fact that we are holding a commitment through prayer.

Health

Prayer for Creative Thought in Health

This prayer is for those who are ill and wish to infuse the healing mantra within. It brings awareness to the connections between body and mind. It encourages the development of faith in our protective forces and the power of our mind.

To be recited morning and evening (or more if desired) during the period of treatment and convalescence.

Prayer for Creative Thought in Health

Magic thought or illusory thought
My thought is my faith
No longer entangled within my mind
My thought turns towards my heart
I receive this thought of love, peace, and healing

Settled deep within my heart, it radiates
It communicates with my organs
That the energy of my body is stable and pure

I no longer need to worry
For the Universe acts for me
It maintains the purity of the conductive threads
And nourishes each of my organs

My body no longer produces
Anything unnecessary for its harmonious
functioning
I am sound in mind and body

Prayer for Preserving Health

This prayer is used for preventing. It is intended for anyone wishing to preserve excellent health.

To be recited regularly once a day for a period of ten days. To be renewed every month. The protocol must be adapted to each person according to their feelings.

Let us remember that the strength of a prayer lies in repetition. Reciting it once will therefore have less impact than when repeated several times with awareness.

Prayer for Preserving Health

Impalpable energies
May you strive
For my body and mind
To function in harmony
Forgetting restraint
And limits

Vaporous spirit
Awakened biochemistry

I am a fortunate being
Who understands all
Today I give thanks
For the balance and life coursing through me

Prayer for Pain

This short prayer is for anyone experiencing acute or aching pain. It can also serve as a mantra for any chronic pain.

To be recited as many times as necessary.

Prayer for Pain

Masters of the unknown Universe and benefactors
Act on my behalf

May from the anvil's might,
Pain become a feather's flight

Prayer to Optimize
a Surgical Procedure

This prayer can be used by anyone facing a surgical procedure. It helps optimize the quality of care and chances of recovery.

To be recited morning and evening in the days leading up to the scheduled surgery. During the surgery, leave a photo of the person inside the prayer book in a dedicated place of recollection. Resume the prayer once the surgery has been completed, at least twice a day in the morning and evening, or more if necessary, until recovery.

Prayer to Optimize
a Surgical Procedure

Masters of Healing, angels of support
With absolute trust my body
Undergoing surgery for (describe or name
the surgery)
To you I entrust without fail
For I am venerable and lack control

Shower me with your presence
For a successful surgery
In the delightful acceptance
Of each of my cells

May my recovery shine
Beneath the blazing healing of the sun

Transform me from body to spirit
From heart to soul
For all is connected to All

Prayer for the Health of a Loved One

This prayer will be beneficial to anyone desiring to wish good recovery to a loved one.

To be recited throughout the duration of the treatment and recovery, once a day. During the rest of the day, place inside the prayer book a photo of the patient and have a white candle lit nearby as often as possible.

Prayer for the Health of a Loved One

O friends of the Universe
Today, I need you close to
(name of the person)
Who suffers from (name the ailment)

With your magic hands
Let energy flow freely

Release the barriers
So the continuous stream of life
Can find its blossoming path

Illuminate the lanterns of healing
Wave the flags that call for help

(name of the person) needs you
To rediscover their unique song

I thank you for your presence
Active and reassuring
And I commend myself to you
With trust and love

Prayer for the Circulation of Fluids (Activation of the Heart Chi)[1]

This prayer and the following exercises are intended for anyone whose health is weakened by a toxic environment, preventing vital fluids from flowing freely. It allows the circuits to be restored through the activation of the heart chi.

To be recited morning and evening throughout the time of discomfort.

To stimulate the heart chi:

– On the heart chakra, between both breasts, place a few drops of vegetable oil[2] mixed with three drops of mandarin essential oil. Take a few moments to soak in this delightful scent.

– Sit or lie comfortably.

– Lengthen your spine.

– Open your heart by straightening your shoulders.

– Place your right hand on your belly (on the navel) and your left hand on your heart.

– Inhale deeply, filling your lungs and belly (count to 5).

– Hold the breath (count to 2).

– Exhale slowly (count to 5).

– Repeat this cycle at least five times.

---

1. [PN] Chi is an imperceptible fluid that creates and animates the universe and all forms of life in Asian cultures.
2. [PN] Sweet almond oil is well-suited for this procedure but can be replaced by any type of vegetable oil, including virgin olive oil.

Prayer for the Circulation of Fluids
(Activation of the Heart Chi)

Heavenly physician, guardian and awakener
Assist my fluids and flows
Into regulation

Perfect pulsation in the tunnels confined
Fluids grant me flexibility so my body is aligned

Help me dissolve the patches
Withdraw the waste
So my body may breathe at its own pace

Guide me along the paths of peace
Where no obstructions shall hinder my journey

I surrender myself into your hands
With all my love

Prayer for Miracles

This prayer serves as a safe summoning upon the unseen forces that work tirelessly towards the improvement of humanity. For the person reciting this intention, it represents an act of unwavering faith accompanied by complete surrender. The occurrence of a miracle won't necessarily happen; it manifests when all conditions align perfectly for the person in question.

To be recited twice a day (or more if necessary), while holding the person in need firmly in your thoughts. Throughout the day, place a photo of the afflicted person inside the prayer book, with a glowing white candle nearby as often as possible.

Prayer for Miracles

Take in first all understandings
Trust in the intelligence of life
Take in with certainty that there's a logic
Trust in not sensing it all
Is your request right?

You may now pray
For the aura of light to embrace you
Or to embrace (name of the person)

Through the strength of this intention
Masters, guides, and protectors
Grant me this miracle
May your arrow of love and truth
Shot with the utmost precision
Reach the evil
To disintegrate, annihilate, transform it

May all the armies of good
Light their torches in unison
Heal me (or heal... name of the person)
From what causes suffering
And whisper in my ears
Wise counsel
So this journey isn't in vain
So it leads to emergence
To openness and clarity

Prayer for Harmful Energies

This prayer is recommended for persons who feel weakened, liable, or in a state of submission regarding a toxic relationship.

It allows them to reclaim their own energy. Parasitic energies are deemed harmful as they do not belong to oneself. Thus, through the power of intention, the person summons forth the best forces.

To be recited slowly, absorbing each word, at least twice a day until a sense of well-being is restored.

Prayer for Harmful Energies

O you, pure source, luminous and radiant
You who animate my being
You who are the breath

Incorporate my being with all your power
Incorporate my mind with all your presence
Let no other power infiltrate

You are light, joy, and the strength of truth
You are the One, the sensitive, and love

You bloom each being
And do not let weeds overcome you
You are the One, joy, and love
The only energy
That my body and mind need

I welcome you within me and repel all others
You are the One, joy, and love

I cling only to you
Savior and healer come from eternity

Prayer to Enhance
the Preparation of Treatment

This prayer is intended to strengthen the effectiveness of treatments and insufflate the intention of healing. It is addressed to doctors, therapists, as well as anyone wishing to optimize the chances of success of their treatment.

If the size of the medications allows, it is possible to place them inside the prayer book throughout the time of treatment. To be recited immediately for any irregular treatment. Can be used at home or in the hospital.

Prayer to Enhance
the Preparation of Treatment

Elixir of Life
Potion of divine love
Be the nectar
Be the miracle

Multiply your power through grace
And generate vibrant healing waves

Every patch of skin or mucous
Every cell is listening to you
And fills with your beneficent energy

Spiritual Growth

Prayer for the Dawning Day

This prayer is intended to awaken the soul when starting a new day. It allows one to fill oneself with positive energies, to surrender to the highest spheres, and to give thanks.

To be recited in the morning once awoken, facing the Sun or toward the rising sun if it is not visible.

Prayer for the Dawning Day

O precious day in rising
Welcome my awakened being
Illuminate my body and soul
With your invigorating energy

Allow me to fulfill the divine will
Through my thoughts, words, and deeds

May my being be open
To the flow of the Source
With confidence and surrender

Everything has a direction
And I take the path
That is most just

Prayer to Regain Faith, Energy

This prayer is to be recited by anyone who feels destabilized, shaken in their beliefs, having lost confidence in themselves and in life. It allows one to cling to divine energy to regain meaning and vitality in life.

To be recited morning and evening for a minimum of ten days. Repeat if necessary.

Prayer to Regain Faith, Energy

O celestial clarity
You who bring forth life
Your strength spreads within me
Floods me and channels me
It ignites my thoughts
Sowing joy and love

Restore my faith in your power
Allow me to heal from what must die
For it is not you, it is not I

Protect me from the dark abysses
Bring me closer to the saving shore
Place before me the beacons of wisdom
And break the pact of illusion
So that I may finally exist

Give me the courage to draw from you
The oxygen of life
Surround me firmly with your enchanting arms
I find refuge only in you

I fully deserve your care
I accept that your enthusiastic energy
Induct peace within me
Thank you

Prayer for the Strength of Will, Determination (Kidney Chi Activation)

This prayer and the accompanying exercises are for anyone wishing to strengthen their will and determination. It activates the kidney chi.

To be recited in the morning once awoken until a sense of improvement is felt.

To stimulate kidney chi:

– Massage the soles of the feet with a few drops of vegetable oil and three drops of mountain rosemary and laurel essential oil.

– Sit on the edge of a chair.

– Lean slightly forward and place your hands above the kidneys, fingers along the spine. You should feel your thumbs below the last ribs.

– Inhale deeply through the kidneys as if you were trying to move your hands. The entire abdominal area is expanded.

– Exhale while emptying the air.

– Perform the exercise for two to three minutes.

Prayer for the Strength of Will, Determination
(Kidney Chi Activation)

Invisible forces of power
Endow me with your unwavering tenacity
Transform me from limp
To unshakable

Prayer for Clear Vision
(Liver Chi Activation)

This prayer and the accompanying exercises are recommended when one seeks to gain more accurate perceptions of situations. Those who immerse themselves in it are committed to being as effective as possible in their analysis, while submitting their judgment to the Source.

To be recited morning and evening, keeping the situation in mind. Stop as soon as the vision is clear and decisions begin to emerge.

To stimulate liver chi:

– Apply a few drops of vegetable oil mixed with three drops of angelica essential oil under the ribs, envisioning a clear and pleasant landscape on the said area.

– Breathe calmly.

– Perform the following breathing exercise (standing or sitting if familiar with the exercise), stare at a specific spot a few feet ahead.

– Inhale deeply through the nose and belly.

– Exhale sharply while controlling your breath, as if releasing an arrow at your target; take power from the abdomen, not the lungs or neck.

– Wait for the next breath to arise spontaneously while remaining relaxed, repeating the exercise four times.

The entire session can be repeated three times as desired.

Prayer for Clear Vision
(Liver Chi Activation)

Combative soul
Cease to struggle for evanescence
Take your stance and pray

O, wondrous Universe
Ancestral wisdom
I connect with you
So you may grant me discernment

My keen sight
Tears through the veil of illusion

The panorama of truth faces me
May each vision be yours
True to the divine plan
Guide me into recognizing
The seductive attire
Of fear and distorted interpretation
May my insight be my arrow

Prayer for Developing Intuition

This prayer is suitable for anyone wishing to develop their intuition and acuity in perceiving intangible elements.

To be recited morning and evening for a period of ten days. Repeat if needed.

Prayer for Developing Intuition

Heaven and Earth unite as one
Above and below are brethren
My mind knows no bounds

Limitless information reaches me
I place my hand
Upon the luminous rail

O easing angels, ensure my protection
Keeping at bay
Strayed souls and other parasites
In the orchestra of my being

It remains to tune the heart
Like a reliable compass
It will guide me
With accuracy and rectitude

Prayer for Wise Choices

This prayer is suited for those who feel hesitant, unsure of their abilities to make choices. It fosters clarity and sets aside the ego.

To be recited twice a day as long as the feeling of indecision persists.

Prayer for Wise Choices

Guides from the celestial world above
Angels of kindness and generosity
I stand by your side
To listen

Help me recognize myself
With insight

Help me choose
The best path

Help me embrace
All possibilities
With reason but without regrets

May this choice align
With the laws of the Universe
To uplift my being
And aid in its fulfillment

Thank you

Prayer for Grounding and Concentration

This prayer is for anyone experiencing difficulties with grounding or concentration. It helps stabilize and restore the ability to adapt better to the environment. It can be widely used with children who have problems concentrating.

To be recited in the morning upon waking for a mindful start to the day. Repeat until symptoms have eased.

Prayer for Grounding and Concentration

May my mind cease racing
Let it settle on its throne
Master of its turmoil
Calm and present to the world

I listen and observe
All my senses awoken

I follow the tracks of perseverance
I drive the train of endurance
and constancy
To reach the station of my goals

Feelings

Prayer for Emotions

This prayer is intended for persons who are naturally emotional or momentarily shaken by a situation. It allows one to accept of the state of imbalance at first, and then to departure from the paths of complaint.

To be recited morning and evening during periods of heightened sensitivity or during an unpleasant situation. Repeat as many times as necessary until a sense of well-being is restored.

Prayer for Emotions

Celestial angel, master of peace
What is this turmoil that roars within me?
I have strayed away from my infinite condition
The one that holds knowledge in all things

I need to realign myself
To reconnect with the soul
That inhabits this bodily space

I am not the thought, swift and impulsive
I am wisdom, temperance

Illuminate every corner of my mind
With your lanterns of clarity
So that I do not confuse ego with truth
Unwind with me
The tendrils of anger, sadness, or resentment
For they ensnare my soul and stifle it

I need you, precious angel
To reveal to myself my mistakes
The emotions I feel
Are but an interpretation
Others would play this role quite differently
So, I choose to listen to your voice
Your voice to speak for me

Prayer for Sadness

This prayer is effective for anyone experiencing a bout of sadness or temporary depression. It restores confidence.

To be recited as many times as desired during times of turmoil (at least twice a day, morning and evening).

Prayer for Sadness

My body is filled with sorrow
Wailing, wandering
In the forgotten limbo of my heart
The abyss is vast, the walls too polished
You once told me
"More than anything do not sink"

Grant me vital momentum
To heal my wounded soul
Support me like an unchanging friend
Unwavering divine grace

Take care of me
In this troubled moment
Light up the steps before me
Upon which I shall tread
Towards renewal

Prayer for Fear

This prayer is to be used by anyone experiencing feelings of fear. It helps to regain calm and peace. It can also be used with children, because even though it may be difficult to understand, the words still play their healing role.

To be recited immediately or once a day if there is a diffuse feeling. Repeat as often as needed until a sense of well-being is restored.

Prayer for Fear

Fear grips me
It overwhelms me
Reduces me to nothing
What is its message?
What truth does it want me to see?

In my inner world
I take refuge
A protective and solid dome
Defines my spaces

O marvelous guides of the infinity
Rein in my wandering mind
Command it to sit still
And contemplate humanity

I pause and position
On the screen of my future
The beginnings of metamorphosis

Prayer Against Jealousy

This prayer is for anyone struggling with feelings of jealousy. It helps to put things into perspective and project thoughts of love.

To be recited when the heart clenches, with full awareness. If the discomfort is pervasive, increase prayers to twice a day. Stop when the feeling of jealousy has disappeared.

Prayer Against Jealousy

O master of wisdom
My being is fragmented
Jealousy gnaws at me
And I cannot find myself

The narrow labyrinth
Twists its infernal coils
And the exit escapes me

My vision is distorted
My thoughts are arrested
I long to leave this emotional prison

Allow me to take flight
To observe and channel
To explore this blooming land
Of my purest feelings

Prayer for Detachment
(for Persons)

This prayer is intended for persons who are unable to feel detached from a relationship. It helps to refocus and channel one's energy towards other goals.

To be recited twice a day, with the aid of a photo of the person alone if necessary. Repeat as often as needed.

Prayer for Detachment
(for Persons)

My Father, my source of life
Through this prayer, I ask for your help
To detach myself from the one
Who has anchored me to him/her

Their ropes are tight
But with your help, I can break free
To regain full control of myself

He/She no longer controls my life
Nor my thoughts
He/She is an individual

Taking flight to other spheres
other relationships
And I, I connect to you to merge
I keep within me only the best
The memories that I nurture

I water only the flowers of happiness
To create a joyful space for myself
The rest flies away with this prayer
And light fills the space that is freed

I am at one with myself
I am proud of myself and my accomplishments
I can function
Relying on my powerful internal resources

Thank you

Prayer for Detachment
(for Situations)

This prayer is for those who find themselves entangled in a situation that seems inescapable. Despite all efforts to detach themselves from it, it continues to instill within them negative thoughts and suffering behaviors.

To be recited twice a day with mindfulness until a better state concerning the situation is achieved.

Prayer for Detachment
(for Situations)

My Father, my source of life
With this prayer I ask for your help
To detach myself from this situation
(briefly describe the situation)
That has anchored itself to me

Their ropes are tight
But with your help, I can break free
To regain full control of myself

It no longer controls my life
Nor my thoughts
I connect with you to merge

I water only the flowers of happiness
To create a joyful space for myself
The rest flies away with this prayer
And light fills the space that is liberated

I am at one with myself
I am proud of myself and my accomplishment
I can function
Relying on my powerful internal resources

Thank you

Prayer to Untangle
a Conflictual Relationship

This prayer is intended for anyone who feels trapped in a con-flictual situation. Through these words, a deep desire to engage in a relationship of respect and peace is expressed.

To be recited twice a day, morning and evening, visualizing the person involved or with the help of their photo, until the conflict is resolved.

Prayer to Untangle
a Conflictual Relationship

Whom do I see? What do I see?
May I rise above
And exile myself for a moment
To discover deep within myself
The reasons behind passion

Is it possible to share
Doubts, anger, resentment?
Is it conceivable to infuse them with a bit of love?

My will is to cultivate in my heart
Compassion, understanding, and discernment

Like an eagle busy in pursuit
I pursue my goal
Which is not to hurt
While knowing how to express myself

Dear divine protections
May from fleeting thoughts
My resolutions clear a path
Of comfort and peace

Stages of Life

Prayer for Welcoming a New Soul

This prayer is for anyone wishing to usher a birth into the best possible circumstances. It allows for the welcoming and protection of the child.

To be recited in the morning at one's convenience and pace.

Prayer for Welcoming a New Soul

A new soul
In the sparkle of life
Has chosen to take seed
Like a new sunrise,
A long-awaited joyful spring

May these new trembling cells
Beat in unison
Welcoming to Earth
A tiny little being

May divine protections
Open their silk parachutes
For a golden and colorful existence

The eternal guild of devoted angels
Rolls out its welcome carpet
And ignites, one by one
The enchanting lights of love

Prayer for Stages of Childhood

This prayer is for parents wishing to help their children through different stages of childhood. It allows acceptance and self-transcendence to grow safely.

To be recited once when waking, during times of turmoil. The child's photo can be placed inside the prayer book during the day.

Prayer for Stages of Childhood

I'm growing
Soon I'll be a man (or a woman)
See how I stretch, how I soar
Help me overcome the rocks
And invincible mountains
Help me cross
The quivering lakes
The untamable oceans
Open with me the chest of untold treasures
Tell me again about the wonders within me

Within me flows the source of happiness
Trumpeting in its arrogant turmoil
How valorous and abundant I am

I'm crossing life's stages
I'm confident and reassured

Prayer for Teenagers

This prayer is intended for anyone wishing to assist a teenager in progressing through the stages of evolution towards adulthood. The teenager themselves can recite this prayer in moments of doubt and confusion.

To be recited in the morning throughout the duration of the disturbance. A photo of the teenager in question can be placed inside the prayer book for the rest of the day.

Prayer for Teenagers

A decisive stage in my changing body
My landmarks shift
And I no longer recognize myself
Sometimes effervescent, sometimes curled up
I await for the change within me
Of the pillars of my life
I need strength and boldness
I don't always know how to express
So listen to the timid song of my heart
May you offer it in echo
The harvest of your experiences
I call out who I am
I don't know who answers

In this overwhelming adventure
Place your jewels of love
To give me peace and stability

Prayer for a Peaceful Menopause

This prayer is highly effective in aiding women crossing the paths of menopause. It offers a different perspective on this transition and restores confidence in one's sacred femininity.

To be recited in moments of disturbance, in the morning, for as many days as desired.

Prayer for a Peaceful Menopause

My call will not go unanswered

Your presence like soft steps of angels
Accompanies me in this moment of transition
My body changes, sometimes rebels
Leading me to unknown tracks
Disturbing my vulnerable mind
Yet I hear the message
of this second spring
Pointing me towards a new path

You whisper
That new worlds are opening up to me
I hear you

Help me on this path of adaptation
Help me to shake off
The projections of a misinformed society

Menopause is not death
It is the opportunity finally seized
To release my glorified energy
To wear my crown of wisdom
To offer my knowledge in sharing

May the discomforts cease
In understanding
And accompanying my being

May joy exist
In love
And solidarity for every being

Prayer for a Better Life in Old Age

This prayer is intended for anyone entering old age. It instills energy and confidence. It can be used in elderly care or retirement facilities.

To be recited upon request, to reconnect with one's inner self.

Prayer for a Better Life in Old Age

I take care of my age
For within it alone
It holds the pearls of my rosary
Sat on the bench of my old age
I hang in the heavens
The sparkling stars of my past

May I have the wisdom to wait and listen
May I not regret
And settle with all my soul
Into the gentle armchair of serenity

My pains, my limits
I offer them to you
So that in return may arise within me
Unexpected desires

Allow me to reach the heights
Conscious and resolute
So that from up there
I perceive the lanterns
Of eternal light

Professional Life

Prayer for Vocation

This prayer is to be used by anyone who is uncertain about their path of fulfillment and wishes to align with the desires of their soul. It helps to secure paths of reflection and to free intuition in order to trust it.

To be recited once a day in the morning during the desired period.

Prayer for Vocation

Like a quivering flower ready to bloom
I seek my path
From my destiny's call

Rain down upon me
Drops of discernment

Close the umbrellas
So that I may watch

Each raindrop
Reflects a message
The one you have for me
To fulfill my vocation to the fullest

Thank you

Prayer to Dedicate a Project

This prayer is intended for anyone eager to place a project under the sign of success.

To be recited at the project's launch or throughout its process as desired.

Prayer to Dedicate a Project

May this project
Auspiciously come to fruition
And receive the blessing it deserves
May it be guided by
Recognition
Success
Prosperity

The Realm Beyond

Prayer for Final Moments

This special prayer is intended for anyone present during the last moments before a soul departs. It allows them to act in the moment to help the soul realize that it is leaving Earth, guiding it towards the best stages of evolution.

To be recited in the moments following the passing, slowly, as many times as the accompanying person deems necessary.

Prayer for Final Moments

It's the moment of the final guard
To acknowledge the passing

Graceful soul surrendered to its departure
See how you are escorted

You fade, you soar
And in the arms of those who love you
The scents of eternal love emerge

Feel how everything is different
Yes, you are free from your chains

From the shackles of your body
Yet you still exist

See how the sky is vast
Hear the praise of the angels and rest
You must acknowledge that you have passed
Passed from a body that lost its use
But whose soul is so rich

You are light, so light
Yet so present
Remain conscious despite the changes

Absorb the transformation
You experience death
Like butterflies experience metamorphosis

You forget your body
But your soul remains intact
You forget your land
But you keep the memory of your loved ones

Everything is calm now
Everything is silent
You bathe in the brilliant and gentle light

Prayer for Accompanying the Passing

This invaluable prayer is a gift offered to the passing person. It serves as genuine guidance, like the comforting hand of an adult enveloping that of a frightened child. It guides the path towards the light and the best supportive entities. It is intended for anyone in contact with someone who is dying and wishes to aid them to passing peacefully.

To be recited in the final moments, with or without the person, as many times as desired. This prayer gains power when performed with several people in a soft, gentle atmosphere scented with candles and incense. Some people appreciate sacred music. Create the reassuring environment that suits them best.

Prayer for Accompanying the Passing

Guides, angels, archangels
Traveling souls of luminous spheres
Whatever your nature
Wherever your horizons
I implore you insistently
To take care of (name of the person)

I pray that you embrace this soul
With all your love
May it be a thousand times powerful

A thousand times irresistible
So that the soul of (name of the person)
Is drawn only to the light

Amid the scent of incense
Mingle those of ancient trees
Those that have seen, felt, heard so many stories

May the wisdom of the world, knowing the wheel
Of life and death
Allow (name of the person) to transition
From one to the other
Smoothly, in ecstasy

May all their qualities soar with them
To flourish their soul and future heart

Take them, if it is destiny
Take them to welcoming skies
Leaving behind tears and affections

Take care of them
Take care of this departing soul
I entrust them into your hands
For eternity

Prayer for Souls in Distress

This prayer is to be recited for souls who have passed away under traumatic conditions.

To be spoken slowly but fervently, at nightfall, for thirty days.

Prayer for Souls in Distress

To lock away in the tomb the bitter buds
The aborted flowers
The black suns

To burn in the fire
The invisible dregs of hell
The deleterious actions
The cloaks of selfishness

With this incantation, Great Divine Source
I implore you to aid the soul of (name of the person)
Brave and resolute
So that at each step
They follow the firmament of their redemption
May lightning bolts become stars of fortune

May the void be filled with love
May this soul recharge with divine energy

With this incantation, Great Divine Source
I thank you for watching over
That they never encounter
The infamous beings

I thank you for taking them to the sound
of your sweet melody
For an eternal harmony

Therapists

Prayer for the Beginning of Healing Sessions

This prayer is essential for any therapist or caregiver wishing to start a session. It allows for the creation of a protective bubble for oneself and the patient, and to summon the best energies for the session.

To be recited once before the session, visualizing a bubble of protection and light around oneself, and then around the patient.

Prayer for the Beginning of Healing Sessions

May the Universe be my armor, from the Cosmos to
the Earth
Enveloped in light, I feel
This powerful wall of protection that secures me
May love invade the space
And act for healing

Lord
May this healing bring to (name of the person)
All the strength of recovery
Through your love and constant presence

Amen[3]

---

3. [PN] This word may seem surprising because it does not belong to the era or culture of the Yellow Emperor. When asked about «Amen,» he re-

Prayer for the End of Healing Sessions

This prayer is essential for any therapist or caregiver who has completed a session. It allows for the release of negative energies and ensures that their shield of protection remains intact.

To be recited once after the session, consciously and calmly. Repeat once if the session has been particularly challenging.

Prayer for the End of Healing Sessions

Cosmic energies, earthly energies,
celestial energies,
Unite your forces to regenerate
My soul, my body, and my spirit

Everything must be connected in an efficient and
healthy network
Everything must work on my behalf

I leave it to the Universe to cleanse,
transform and secure
I am only a messenger, a transmitter
I retain no miasma, no attachment

---

sponded that it is necessary to use language that can be understood by those for whom the healing is intended.

Everything is returned to the Universe
To provide to the other what they need

Animals

Prayer for Welcoming an Animal

This prayer is for anyone wishing to ease the welcoming of an animal into their home.

To be recited at the time of welcoming, once a day during the adaptation period.

Prayer for Welcoming an Animal

What is the boundary between it and I?
We may be brothers
(name of the animal) joins our home
And joy embraces our hearts

Thank you for helping us
To love it, to cherish it, to understand it
May our listening
Come from heart and kindness

Men and animals are brothers
May we give to each other
In laughter and complicity
For the elevation of species
On the scale of the Universe

Prayer for a Sick Animal

This prayer is for anyone wishing to improve the health of their animal.

To be recited once a day throughout the duration of the animal's treatment and convalescence. It is also possible to leave a photo of the animal inside the prayer book for the rest of the day.

Prayer for a Sick Animal

O angels of animals
Take care of (name of the animal)
Sick and weakened

Apply your celestial ointments
On its energy-deprived body
Administer the pills of tenderness
So that soon
(Name of the animal) is on its feet
Vigorous and joyful

Places

Prayer for Purifying Places

This prayer is for anyone wishing to purify a space. It clears out lingering toxic energies and restores a pure energy within the area.

Recite it once with the purification protocol. Repeat the entire protocol if necessary.

Purification protocol to perform alongside the prayer:

– Create a smudging bundle with white sage and rosemary.

– Perform sweeping motions with the bundle to move the energies of the space, starting from the corners, then moving in up and down and side to side.

– Leave the room closed until the smoke dissipates.

– Open the windows to ventilate and create airflow if possible. Complete the process by burning resin incense (such as myrrh) to re-energize the space.

– Repeat the process if the space is heavily charged.

Prayer for Purifying Places

No shadow, no reflection
No trace
May this unique place vibrate for itself
Healthy and rid of its indolent parasites
Of its wandering beings

The smoke of healing plants
Encloses the unwanted energies
And heals the wounds
Of worn-out auras

This place pulsates with love
And welcomes me to its altar
For a new journey
With health and protection

Plants

Prayer for the Growth of Plants

This prayer is for anyone sensitive to the well-being of plants. It will help stimulate growth and limit the appearance of diseases or parasites.

To be recited at the time of planting or if the plant is showing signs of weakness.

Prayer for the Growth of Plants

Being, vibrant and awake
Dynamic branches (or stems)

Impatient roots
To propel their living sap

I call upon all subtle energies
To infuse you with health and vigorous growth
So may it be my plan

Table of Contents

9 781913 191443